RUNNER'S DISCOVERY JOURNAL

60 Days To Get Fit and Fired Up To Do Anything

Sara Grace

GRACE
MEMOIRS

New York

CONTENTS

CONTENTS

DAY 1:
DON'T PSYCHE YOURSELF OUT

January 1, 2010: 6.3 miles, 1:10. YT: 6.3 miles. Ran on the beach as far as the power plant at El Segundo. Sluggish at first but finished strong. Saw Kooky Groovy Lady, a leathery late 60's broad who moves down the path, headphones on, like she's grooving at Woodstock. But awkwardly.

DATE: _____ **TIME:** _____ **MILES:** _____

NOTES:

So, it's Day 1. Are you ready? I thought I was ready when I decided to embark on the Thousand Mile Year, my project to run and document a year of running. And yet, once I had built the web site and "locked" myself into it—just as you have with this purchase—it started making me anxious. Commitment-phobia, anyone?

I plunged forward by telling myself what I actually still tell myself before every long run: *Stop thinking and GO!* And so must you.

They say that anything we can imagine, we can do, but when it comes to physical activity (unlike building planes or faster computers or hydrogen engines), you're better off jumping straight to *do.*

Don't try to imagine yourself running nine miles, or, even three, if that's a challenge for you today. If you're like me, it's right up there with imagining cutting your arm off with eyebrow tweezers. Don't GO there. Just get on the road, or the track or the treadmill, and run what little bit you can. It might be 50 minutes, or it might be five.

And if you're going to imagine something, imagine yourself after your daily run—a little bit lighter, and proud of what you've done. *Ready, set... GO!*

JOURNAL SPACE

About your goal: What do you want to have achieved 3 months from now when you're finished with this journal? Write it here, and review it when there's a day you don't feel like running.

DAY 2:
GET ON PROGRAM

January 20, 2010: 4.3 miles, 41 min. YT: 59.9 miles. My first New York run, ever. Also my first run without coffee in I don't know how long. Fortunately the dramatic views of the East River—under the Williamsburg bridge, under the Manhattan Bridge— and very raw wind kept me moving.

DATE: _____ **TIME:** _____ **MILES:** _____

NOTES:

A training program is the perfect companion to the daily "nudge" that this book provides. Here are some of the best training programs available for free online:

• Couch to 5k: Designed to get you running 5 uninterrupted kilometers in 9 weeks, and there's a C25k iPhone App. (See *http://www. c25k.com/*.)

• Hal Higdon's 10K training program: Hal, one of the running world's most famous trainers, offers novice, intermediate, and advanced versions of this 8-week program. (*See (http://www.halhigdon.com/ training/51122/10K-Novice-Training-Program.*)

• Half-marathon (aka Half-Mary, aka Bloody Mary) training program for beginners from Marathon Rookie: This is a 10-week program that assumes you have been running for at least four weeks and can run 30 minutes without stopping before beginning the schedule. (*See http://www.marathonrookie.com/half-marathon-training.html.*)

Finally, if you're feeling spendy, at RunnersWorld.com you can order training programs that are delivered daily by email.

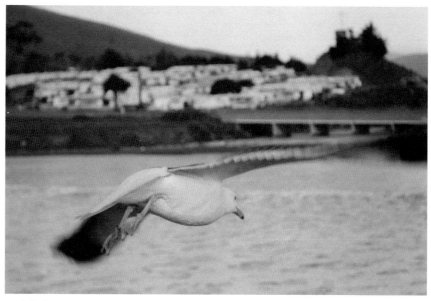

Bird flight in Cayucos, CA, where the 1000MY was launched.

DAY 3:
A FEW ASSIGNMENTS

January 22, 2010: 2.9 miles, 29 minutes. YT: 62.8 miles. Back from NY. My brain was completely empty today. All I can remember is the feel of the rain on my face, the warmth of being overly dressed, and the moment where I could feel my body wake up.

DATE: _____   TIME: _____   MILES: _____

NOTES:

I'm a big believer in not letting a bunch of *shoulds* stand between you and your goal. At some point that kind of to-do list becomes a tool for procrastination and making excuses. On some level, you just need to lace up and get out there. But, look at you, now on Day 3! So since you've already gotten started, here are a few more things I suggest doing to prepare for the road ahead:

• Consider a check up if it's been a while. This seems to be boilerplate advice for every fitness routine every written. So why not? If nothing else, you'll feel like you've taken care of yourself.

• If you haven't already, choose a training plan and block off some regular times that you know work for running. You're much more likely to stick to the plan if you've carved out space for it. Consistency helps.

• Take measurements. If you're doing this even in part to lose weight or improve your physique, this is important because your weight will likely jump up for a few weeks as your muscles respond to this new activity. Measurements will help assure you that your body is still getting smaller, whatever the scale says.

• Think about your feet. Visit a high-end running store and have them evaluate your stride. If you already have a pair of running or athletic shoes, bring them so they can analyze wear.

• Get entrenched. Read *Runner's World* to get a sense of the community and the sport. Then find other runners by joining a site like DailyMile.com. Putting yourself inside a community of other people who are doing what you're doing will keep you focused, even when the rest of the world is constantly saying things like, "6 a.m. runs? Are you *crazy?*"

Again: find time for running first. Getting the rest of this stuff done comes second.

DAY 4:
WHERE TO RUN

January 23, 2010: 6.4 miles, 1:10 minutes. The beach path was almost totally covered in sand. I pushed myself and it felt good. My attempt to enter a meditative state, less successful. My iPod is now only playing in one ear. It outlasted the former fiance who gave it to me by more than three years.

DATE: _____ TIME: _____ MILES: _____

NOTES:

One thing that I love about running is that it helps to make exercise the path of least resistance. You don't have to drive to a gym or pull together a team. You just put on your sneakers (and hopefully some clothes) and go.

So what I recommend is that, if it's at all possible, you run right outside your front door. But I also recommend sunlight, fresh air, and passing scenery. If you have knee or joint problems, get off the pavement to dirt or a track as much as you can. (You might also look into chirunning.com, which helps you learn to run in a way that puts less stress on your body.)

Personally I prefer a route that is part traveling, and part loops. Having a park that you loop around helps me get my stride; something about the repetition keeps me going. At the same time, I think I'd get bored if I didn't also have a few miles of open road.

If your neighborhood isn't good for running, second best is to drive or bike to somewhere that's better.

Third best is the gym. I generally avoid the gym, except for occasional timed runs or controlled hill climbs. But if you love it, more power to you. If you don't love it but have to run in a gym for whatever reason, make the best of it. Buy a membership at the most expensive sweat box you can afford. Get yourself a cute outfit, make friends with the guy at the desk, and pick a time when you're not going to have to wait for a machine. Allay yourself of the steam room and any other awesome extras. On the treadmill, cover the display so you're not constantly ticking off minutes. You want to let your brain run wild (time flies), not be anchored to those numbers (time creeps).

Now, think about your schedule: What is a weekly time slot that you can commit to consistently devoting to a good solid hour of fitness (it doesn't all need to be running), with added time for transportation to somewhere where you know you'll really enjoy it?

DAY 5:
SUFFERING IS OPTIONAL

January 25, 2010: 6 miles, 1:03 minutes. YT: 75.2 miles. GREAAAAAT RUN. Kundalini lady was out in her pink jump suit, flailing her head around, her own special ecstatic brand of davening. Intense bearded man crossed my path three times, and faster than me. Zing.

DATE: _____ TIME: _____ MILES: _____

NOTES:

In yoga, they're always talking about "lubricating the joints" with bends and stretches. After a great run, I feel like every cell of my body has been lubricated. I feel purposeful and clear. I can handle every challenge. Everything else seems relative to my run: That is the ultimate challenge, the real life, the center of things. I feel grounded, and yet completely light. Is this "runner's high?" Endorphins, fairy dust, whatever—it feels good and solid. If you're just starting your running life, you may not feel like this yet, but you will.

My favorite author Haruki Murakami wrote a memoir on running, *What I Talk About When I Talk About Running.* He went from being a chain smoker to being an hour-daily runner so that he could keep his creativity flow strong enough to churn out novel after amazing novel.

I loved this quote:

"This book does contain a certain amount of what might be dubbed life lessons. They might not amount to much, but they are personal lessons I've learned through actually putting my own body in motion, and thereby discovering that suffering is optional."

Put your body in motion.

Suffering. Is. Optional.

These are the mantras of this journal. Let them be the mantras of your run, and your life.

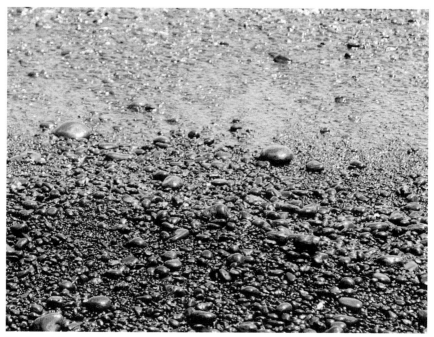

Black rock beach in Hana, Maui.

DAY 6:
MIND, BODY, SPIRIT

January 26, 2010: 3.2 miles, 37 minutes. YT: 78.4 miles. New definition of determina-
tion: The look on the face of the tubby old Chinese lady in Capri pants and sports
flip-flops with socks who comes down Grand View daily in a waddling jog.
I love her.

DATE: _____ TIME: _____ MILES: _____

NOTES:

The transformative power of running is more than inspiration.
As you move from being a nonrunner, or an occasional 3-miler, to
a person who runs 10K as the stretch of a leg (or heaven help me, a
marathon) you are, through discipline and diligence, literally trans-
forming yourself. You will get thinner. Your muscles will get stronger and sleeker. You will have more energy and sleep better. And if
you're me, your hangovers won't be as bad and your blood sugar will
stabilize.

But I'm not talking about a physical transformation so much
as a mental one—and yet they are so closely related it's almost like
staring into a glass of water and trying to see the individual drops.

I started my running believing very strongly that I was not
meant to be a "real" runner. Or at the very least, not a distance run-
ner. We've all got what the self-help crowd calls "limiting beliefs."
If you've always been athletic, yours may manifest somewhere else.
("I'm not creative." "I'd never have the courage." "I can't work the
DVD player.")

Limiting beliefs can be particularly powerful when it comes to
exercise because these beliefs are wrapped up in our physical bod-

ies. I remember as a child always fearing group hikes. Because I was slightly heavier than everyone else, and not particularly athletic, I thought I would be the slowest, the reddest, the huffiest and puffiest.

So guess what? I never tried to lead. I purposely brought up the rear, content with being the straggler. Or I would avoid group athletics. Years later, as an adult with a decade of regular exercise under my belt, I realized one day on a group hike that I was actually among the fittest in the bunch.

Even today, as someone who can run a couple 10Ks a week, there are times that I fight the mental image of myself as someone who's most comfortable, most herself, while at rest. Even today, I have to talk myself out of that mental image sometimes to get my butt running. And, voila, I have still other limiting beliefs to contend with—such as the idea that excess, of food, wine, or fun, is to be celebrated.

Fake it 'til you make it, people. If your body goes through the motions enough, the mind will follow.

JOURNAL SPACE

What's your limiting belief and where does it come from?

DAY 7:
RUN AN HOUR IN 20 MINUTES

January 30, 2010: 6.9 miles, 1:19 minutes. I don't know if it was my rest day yesterday, or eating before, or sleeping nine hours last night, or Lady Gaga remixes, but I had much more energy in the first half of this run than I usually do. Big surf to look at, and two sail boats washed up on shore. Actually, one and a half.

DATE: _____ TIME: _____ MILES: _____

NOTES:

Give your brain something interesting to think about during your run. Otherwise, when you first get started, here's how your mental dialogue will go:

SUFFERING. GRUELING. EXHAUSTION.

SWEATY, SWEATIER, SWEATIEST.

Guaranteed: Your run will feel like the longest 30 minutes of your life.

Instead, give your brain an assignment: Organize your day, ruminate on health care, consider the past three months of your relationship. Make a mental list of important people in your life, and who you need to catch up with. Think about your favorite book. Give a review, Ebert-style, of the last movie you watched.

Just don't think about your run. If you run on a treadmill, I recommend covering up the display so your mind is free to wander. Eventually, when you start working on pacing, you may need some more focus on how you're moving your body through space.

But at the beginning, let your imagination dance.

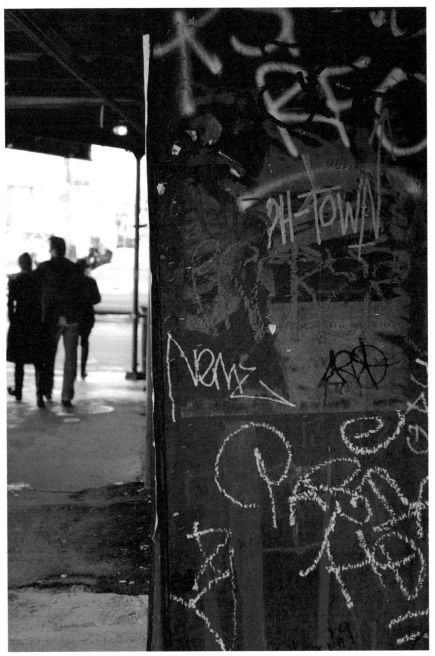

Signs of life. New York City, near 14th St.

DAY 8:
GET A SOUNDTRACK

January 31, 2010: 3.4 miles, 41 minutes. YT: 96.8. That run was like a gymnast trying desperately to make an off-balance backhandspring stick. Except it was a cartwheel and I still fell over at the end. It happens.

DATE: _____ TIME: _____ MILES: _____

NOTES:

Spend some time today putting together an amazing new playlist for your next run. Music is another great way to push past the lazy. Think of your run as a dance, and get swept up in a rhythm that ispires you.

Podrunner.com has a zillion free podcasts (make a donation!), mostly progressive and house music. I like to run with all kinds of music, but there's nothing quite like electronic to pick me up and pull me through a long run. Also, when I download new tracks, it helps me get excited for my next run, when I'll get to hear them.

Here are my top five of the moment, all about an hour long and between 135–155 bpm (on the slow side, but that's how I kick it). The (enjoyably) corny titles and descriptions are Podrunner's:

• *Strong* – mind body heart beats

• *Easygoing* – this one starts out a bit jazzy, moves on to a funky house vibe, and builds to a prog house finish to make your going a lot easier

• *Chants Meeting* – a hypnotic, lulling workout mix that will zone you out and bring you back to earth hardly even aware of the calories you've burned

- *Paradox Alley* – opposites at track
- *Breezy* – An uplifting breath of fresh air that will move you along for nearly an hour

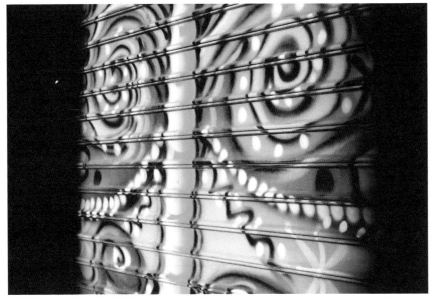

Security door art. New York City, 2010.

DAY 9 :
POST-RUN RECOVERY DRINK

February 12, 2010: 3.8 miles, 44 min. YT: 132.6. Training plan said "easy," I took it easy. As I came down the hill, a favorite song came on and felt just right to the gray day, the mountains hidden completely in clouds and fog, the trees in a dozen shades of muted green. I hit repeat on the Ipod three times.

DATE: _____ TIME: _____ MILES: _____

NOTES:

I ran my first 10K race a few years ago—"run" being a stretch of the term. I shuffled through it, gritting my teeth all the way through. Afterwards, we went to a '50s diner and had shockingly huge breakfasts. Then we went home and collapsed on the couch for the rest of the day. What athletes we were.

These days, I have terrific energy all day after long runs. It's in part being in better shape, but I also chalk it up to my awesome recovery drink. This is what I eat after a run, and I generally wait at least two to three hours before I have my next solid meal. There are many theories on how to handle recovery eating; this is just what works for me. It keeps a spring in my step.

GREEN RECOVERY DRINK
- 1 cup unsweetened almond or coconut milk (whatever level of fat you want; I get the fattiest)
- 1 cup water
- 1 scoop Macro Greens (available online and at Whole Foods)
- 1 scoop Designer Whey Protein ("research proven," but to do

what, we don't know)
- Ice cubes
- ½–1 cup berries or other fruit (optional; I don't usually add fruit, but I will admit it tastes better that way)

Blenderize and drink!

JOURNAL SPACE:

Are you feeding yourself properly? Commit here to a healthy pre- or post-workout eating habit. Try it for a few weeks. See how it works for you. Then tweak.

DAY 10:
SOLIPSISM IS GOOD—FOR RUNNING

February 14, 2010: 10 miles, 1:46 minutes. My last beach run before six weeks of cold in New York, in the most perfect weather of the year so far. Kooky Groovy Lady was out today, in a rhinestone-accented shirt, magenta-acid-washed denim cutoffs, and matching magenta and black sneakers. Thinking about love.

DATE: _____ TIME: _____ MILES: _____

NOTES:

In the big, bad world of running, 1000 miles in a year ain't nothin' special. You feel a perspective shift as you start to inhabit a world where people run a sub 4:00 marathon every month. They all seem so...Athletic. So dedicated. So fit.

So what? In any endeavor—athletic, creative, or otherwise—there's always going to be someone doing it bigger and better than you. But if you're like me, you make the mistake of comparing yourself to others. When you do this, you're sending yourself a negative message: "I'm less. I'm not good enough. I'm not *enough.*" Boy, that can't be motivating, can it? It would mean that every time you run, you're failing just by doing it. Not a good place to be.

So, no judging. Stay focused on exploring your experience. It's yours alone, unique to the world, and that's something. Also, as Walt Whitman famously said, "Great battles are lost in the same spirit they are won." How you throw yourself at the effort is what counts. Keep doing. Doing is playful, animating, reaffirming. Stay still, and risk analyzing your best impulses to death. This applies to more than running.

DAY 11:
ALL TOMORROW'S DISCIPLINE

January 4, 2010: 57 min, 5.15 miles. YT: 17.80. Incredible skies and moon over West LA; the Hollywood Hills and San Gabriels were crisp, but lower to the ground, Hollywood was in a thick yellow smog.

DATE: _____ TIME: _____ MILES: _____

NOTES:

Success lies in setting the prerequisites. You can have all the will in the world, but you've got to lay the practical groundwork along with it. What are you doing to support your fitness program? Try to do at least one of these this week:

• Get adequate sleep.

• Drink less alcohol. (I can only offer second-hand data for the efficacy of this.)

• Eat healthy foods in substantial enough quantities to fuel yourself.

• Lay your running clothes out the night before a run, and make sure they're comfy and you like them. (Buy new togs otherwise.)

• Go to bed knowing exactly when and how long you will run the next day. Setting goals in this way works with your brain's machine language to set yourself up for success.

JOURNAL SPACE

Is there an activity that's sabotaging your running efforts? Identify it here. Consider what need it's serving. Is there something healthier that you can replace it with that will serve the same need?

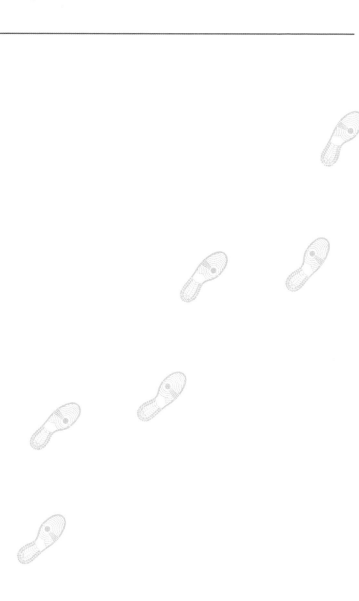

DAY 12:
SHUT UP THE GREMLINS AND RUN

February 26, 2010: 4.1 miles, 42:50 minutes. Today was my first run in the gym, since NYC was a big pile of snow. I saw a woman sink her foot ankle deep in slush. She took it well. Most people were well-suited in galoshes. I picked my way across Union Square in sneakers to head to the gym.

DATE: _____ **TIME:** _____ **MILES:** _____

NOTES:

It's not always easy to pull yourself out of bed, especially if you're facing nasty weather or winter darkness. The gremlins WILL natter in your ear, disguised as your friends and caretakers: *You're tired, dearheart. Running is hard. It's cold out. It's going to be hard and unpleasant. You deserve your rest.*

Unless it's -40 Celsius, and you haven't slept in 24 hours, they're not your friends. Here's how to shut them up:

1. Keep this book on your bedside table, to read pages like this one.

2. Fill your head with thoughts about how you'll feel after the run: *Accomplished. Strong. Fitter. Joyful.*

3. If that's not enough, enlist help: Your iPod. Put your earphones on, right there in bed. Play a song that gets you moving.

4. If that still doesn't work, bargain. Tell yourself, "You don't have

to go running, but you DO have to get up and put on your running clothes." That's all, just get dressed. Then, once you're dressed, tell yourself, "You don't have to run, you just have to leave the house and walk." Leave the house. Nine times out of ten, you'll end up running. And if not, you'll get a good walk in.

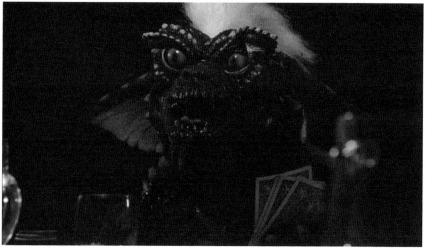

Homage to a dubious '80s classic.

DAY 13:
DO IT YOURSELF

March 8. 2010: 3.14 miles, 32:28 minutes. YT: 187.79. Oscar c"Up"cakes and chardon-nay made for a slow run on a nevertheless incredible morning. The sun shines even on the sluggish.

DATE: _____   TIME: _____   MILES: _____

NOTES:

If you want some crazy thing in this world, you damn well better make it happen yourself. No doubt, you will encounter many caring, supportive people along the way. Success isn't "you vs. the world," but they can't do the job for you. You've got to lead the world to the proper decision about your fate—gorgeous, amazing success.

Case in point: I used to work for this crazy, awesome independent film distribution company. We released films about Ethiopian Jews, films about blackly comic goings-on in cold Icelandic landscapes, films about coups in South America—yeah, you get it: films that no other theatrical distribution company would touch with a 1000 foot pole. And they were great movies, too.

Anyway, my boss hated hiring PR firms. In part it was because we were always broke. But he was also right when he said, "No one is going to work as hard for your movie as you are."

Ultimately, no one is going to make your dreams happen but you. If you're not ready to fight for it—particularly if your idea is innovative or eccentric in any way—it ain't gonna happen.

Likewise with your crazy running regimen, workout plans, commitments to diet and exercise, whatever. If you don't demand the time and the space for your plans from the people in your life, it ain't gonna happen.

Stick your ground, and get on the road!

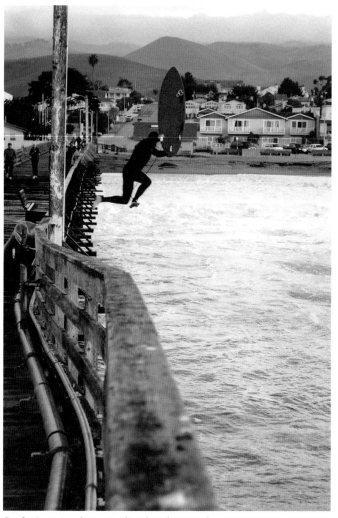

Surfer jumping from pier lined with signs that say "no jumping."

DAY 14:
RUNNING CHIC

March 10, 2010: 4.79 miles, 47:48 minutes. Year total: 192.58. In East River Park, I saw a pair of jeans and a comforter stuffed into the lower limbs of a small tree. I guess it was someone's PJs and bedding—in their "dresser." Hope it's there when he or she goes back tonight.

DATE: _____ TIME: _____ MILES: _____

NOTES:

A conversation I had last week with my coworker:

Me: I definitely think more men look at me from cars when I run wearing lipstick.

Craig: Yeah. They're wondering why you're wearing lipstick to go running.

Lipstick may be overkill, but I absolutely suggest that you wear running clothes that you love, that feel like you—whether it be the color, the design on the shirt, the fit, or the length.

If you feel like a trussed-up chicken in your running togs, your subconscious is (quite reasonably) going to work subtly, consistently, to thwart you.

Make sure your running bra fits, avoid anything that requires contortionism to get into it, and forget any spandex that screams "sausage links" or "muffin top."

If you feel good, and comfortable, always comfortable, in your clothes, you're more likely to feel like running is something you're supposed to be doing.

Enjoy today's run, with or without the lipstick.

DAY 15:
THE RACE OF A THOUSAND TEARS

March 13, 2010: 4.97 miles, 52:04. YT: 200.72. Rain, rain, rain. Cold, cold rain. Hundreds of dripping runners. 10% pleasure in our hard-core devotion; 90 percent WTF am I doing standing in the freezing rain preparing to run 5 miles with a bunch of crazy people?

DATE: _____ **TIME:** _____ **MILES:** _____

NOTES:

Consider signing yourself up for a nearby race—even if you don't feel ready for a bib, just explore the options. Do a Google search so that you know what's out there. Or pick a date to race against yourself, a focused push to complete a certain distance faster than you ever have. It'll fire you up.

My first real race—one that I really trained for—was the New York Road Runners Central Park 8K. It was basically a disaster from beginning to end: I got to the starting line 45 minutes early because I was so afraid I'd be late, and then stood for an hour in freezing rain in Central Park before the gun went off.

Still, what I liked about the experience:

• Experiencing the camaraderie of the craziness of the whole frozen, wet endeavor with fellow runners. I still haven't known a nastier day of weather in NYC.

• Knowing that I was capable and prepared—obviously not to win, but to run "my race."

• Running in a pack, when I'm used to solitary runs.

• Finally having a race T-shirt, and in my favorite color.

What I didn't like:

• Having to pick up my bib at 6:30 a.m.

• Being numb and soaked by the time the race started.

• Being numb again two minutes after the race had ended.

• The fact that my Nike Plus was totally inaccurate, so that I ran a much slower race than I thought I had, despite what felt like maximum effort.

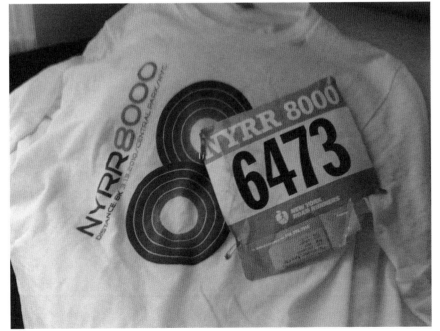

Love the race shirt, hated the race.

DAY 16:

WHY DO YOU RUN?

March 16, 2010: 2.1 miles, 20-something minutes. YT: 202.73 miles. Treadmill run and pilates. Trying to get my body back in balance after a heinous case of dry eyes. But the weather in NY turned warm and sunny again, and there were people playing soccer in Union Square Park when I walked home at 10:30 at night. NY and I have both turned a corner.

DATE: _____ TIME: _____ MILES: _____

NOTES:

Are you running to run away from something? Is running just the healthy version of drinking, a cloud of endorphins replacing a tipsy glow?

Maybe. But at least when we're ready to do the work of healing, we're healthy and strong, not hungover and cranky.

And so, my answer to the question, "Why do you run?"—or at least to why I started running: To get over a break up, of course. Why else?

Well, more or less.

It was actually six months after my "official" breakup, but if you've ever been in a serious long-term relationship, you know that ending things isn't like crossing the bridge from the US to Mexico. It's a long, painful transatlantic flight to Siberia. It takes time.

Come September 2009, I had landed in Siberia, alone. I was frustrated and lonely, and ready to throw myself at the world. The solution was to spend too much time at a bar called Hal's, drinking white wines from New Zealand and kissing inappropriate men under the shadows of palm trees and street lamps.

In the mornings, I'd drag my mildly (or occasionally excrutiatingly) hungover body out of bed. Sometimes I did something I had never done before: I smoked cigarettes before breakfast. Sometimes four. I'd crawl to the kitchen, make coffee, and absorb myself in meaningless Internet until my boss started Skyping me, then I'd absorb myself in whatever work demanded.

I rarely felt good. I felt every part of me hardening up like an orange that dries as it's rotting.

I realized quickly that I had evolved into a situation that threatened to become damaging, to my body, my heart, my work, and my future relationships.

And I realized that if I was to change directions, I needed another path to walk on.

Or, at it turned out, to run on. Running was my way out. I ordered a *Runner's World* training series, which doubled the amount of miles I had previously been running and introduced speed work, something I'd never done before. Very quickly I began to feel better. Grounded. Whole.

Maybe it's better not to ask what you're running from, but what you're running toward. Understand the "why" behind your desire to run, and you'll find a deeper well of motivation than you've ever known before.

JOURNAL SPACE

Being healthy is a great end goal, but ask yourself another question: What do you want all that radiant health, beauty, and energy to enable you to do? What big goals (1 year +) do you have on your plate? They could be as dramatic as launching a business, or as personal as having more energy to be a mother or friend.

DAY 17:
A TASTY RECIPE

March 20, 2010: 5.8 miles, 1 hr, 3 min. YT: 211.53. I drank wine up and down Avenue A last night, and paid for it with this slow, slow run along the East River. There were four people fishing today. Hopefully just for sport?

DATE: _____ **TIME:** _____ **MILES:** _____

NOTES:

If you haven't tightened up your diet, maybe today's the day to start. My preferred diet is close to what is generally referred to these days as "paleo": mostly vegetables, animal proteins, and fat. My carbs average 100–150 grams a day, when I'm eating my cleanest. If you are interested in trying low-carb or paleo eating, I highly recommend MarksDailyApple.com, and all of Mark's books, as best in class. But it's clear to me that everyone's body is different, so if you're a vegan or a fruitarian or an ovolactarian or a pescatarian and it's working for you, keep at it.

Whatever you were eating in the past, however, you're now eating to fuel several runs a week, so you might need to make changes. Start paying attention: Which foods are helping, which are hurting? Experiment. See what makes you feel best. Replace the bad with the good.

Your body will show you the way.

If you're looking for new ideas, here's one of my favorite quick weeknight meals—one of the few vegetarian meals I eat regularly these days:

TEMPEH WITH BROCCOLI

1 block tempeh (I don't do too much soy, but tempeh I like)

1 bag or head of broccoli

1 tsp or so sesame oil

2 cloves garlic or large shallot, minced

SAUCE:

1-2 tbsp. peanut butter

1 tsp. honey (optional; to taste)

couple tsp. hot sauce

couple tbsp. soy

couple tbsp. white wine or rice vinegar

2 tsp. (or so) minced ginger

DIRECTIONS:

1. Saute tempeh in a tsp or two of sesame oil with garlic or shallot (careful not to burn!).

2. Make sauce. You may want to double the volumes above the first time and see how much you like.

3. Add broccoli to tempeh pan and drizzle sauce over.

4. Add a little water if needed to keep it from being too dry.

5. Add lid for a superquick steam.

6. Open and saute if needed until broccoli is cooked but firm. Should still be bright green!

Enjoy!

DAY 18:
NEVER RUN ALONE—SOMETIMES

March 22, 1010: 2.4 miles, 27:27 minutes. Today's run continued the day's trend of
agonizing about whether to move to NY permanently. Endless listing of pros and
cons. Poking and prodding at the intangibles of happiness. Finally, after running,
weights, a steam, and a short walk in a beautiful rainy night, a little bit of peace.
Life is a gift.

DATE: _____   TIME: _____   MILES: _____

NOTES:

"In this day of the Internet, no one ever goes through anything alone," a writer commented in an article in *The New York Times* about an over-50 Dads' support group.

So true! And so helpful, when you consider this quote from Christakis and Fowler's book, *Connected*, that shows how much a community can affect you: "Happiness is more contagious than unhappiness...each additional happy friend boosts your good cheer by 9 percent, while each additional unhappy friend drags you down by only 7 percent." Turns out friends are a winning proposition. Who knew?

I highly recommend you find some happy, running friends in the online running community DailyMile.com, if you haven't already. There, you can log daily training, meet other runners in your area, and just generally get a little whiff of runner's high without leaving your computer.

DAY 19:
SELF CHECK-IN

March 24, 2010: 5 miles, 52:11 minutes. I'm rounding down the mileage number these days to correct for NikePlus inaccuracy of my apparently wild, unmeasurable gait. Today I ran on a track. The monotony of it, and the smoothness of the terrain, is relaxing. Plus it's fun to be on a course with other runners.

DATE: _____ **TIME:** _____ **MILES:** _____

NOTES:

Writing down your training program makes you a much better runner—you're focused on progress, moving from A to a B, not just "working out." Are you looking to increase distance or speed or both? You decide.

A plan keeps you honest. It also gives you a chance to WIN everytime you follow through on a workout.

Now, if you're faithfully following the advice in this book, you're already on a plan—bravo! Today, review it and decide whether you've got it right. Check in with yourself: How's your body doing? Is it time to increase your mileage or speed? Can you safely push yourself a little harder than you thought you could? Or are you pushing yourself too hard?

You only get one body. Take care of it!

DAY 20:
MY PET FARTLEK

March 27, 2010: 5.96 miles, 1:03. YT: 224.89 miles. Soooo cold and miserable. Felt OK otherwise. I saw a little red tug boat pulling a barge on the East River! I felt a kinship with it, me pulling my reluctant body along.

DATE: _____ TIME: _____ MILES: _____

NOTES:

Earlier I wrote about how to make an hour long run feel like 20 minutes. That post could have equally been about the Fartlek. Ah, Fartlek. How I love thee.

For new runners, a quick explanation: A Fartlek is an interval workout. It means "speed play" in Swedish, the nationality of the coach who invented it to train cross-country runners. It's the perfect name, because it's actually a super fun run to do—you know, "playful." The way you ran when you were a kid.

During the intervals, you use your own level of exuberance to determine your fast speed. Liberating, no? It actually makes me run faster since my speed is a choice, not something I have to do. I get very antsy about things I perceive as "duties."

I also like Fartlekking (so much so I'm inventing the gerund form) because it produces the "afterburn" associating with interval training—your metabolism gets a kick that continues for hours after your run.

Here was one of my Fartlek runs:

• 15 minutes easy.
• 1 minute hard, one minute easy x 5.

- 10 minutes of easy running.
- 1 minute hard, one minute easy x 5.
- 10 minutes of easy running

The fast intervals are the most fun part of the run. You may not feel quite like a kid again, but at least like a speedy cartoon character adult. Wheeeeeeee!

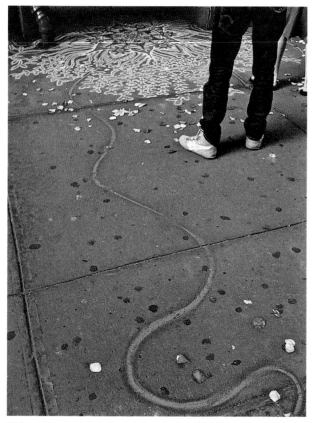

Sidewalk art on 19th Street, for playful spirits.

DAY 21:
TO RUN IS TO LIVE

April 11, 2010: 5.9 miles, 1:07 minutes. YT: 349.5. Three trendy hipster teens walking together over the bridge reminded me of Desperately Seeking Susan. *One was in black floral lace stockings with short-shorts. And they all had the attitude.*

DATE: _____ TIME: _____ MILES: _____

NOTES:

Running brings a particular physical and mental high that I enjoy. But I also love that it's a great metaphor for life. You plan your run, you run it, you push yourself, you slack, you stumble, you leap. And eventually you return to where you started. It doesn't mean anything at all in the grand scheme of the universe, or even to the people who live next door to you. But it means something to you. And if you're lucky, to the small circle of people who care about the air you're breathing.

After I finish running, I feel like giving someone a sweaty, knock-'em-down hug. That's a great feeling to bring to the world.

DAY 22:
GRATITUDE RUN

April 20, 2010: 3.7 miles. 39:37 minutes. YT: 269.7 miles. Great, great run. I worked myself into a frenzy replaying the gentle yelling match I had with Umberto, my building super who is at war with the younger residents of the building.

DATE: _____ **TIME:** _____ **MILES:** _____

NOTES:

If you've got one of those bodies that seems to be preparing for famine every time you put something in your mouth, you may feel cursed. You've probably had at least some period of *why me?-dom*, and maybe you regularly end up eating things you shouldn't be-cause in those moments of self-pity, you think that since the world made you fat, then you at least deserve some delicious cheesecake. Take that, world! And can I please have some more?

Hopefully you don't have any of these problems. Hopefully you were born hating cheesecake. But for the rest of us, let's flip it. What if you started to think about your struggle with extra poundage as a blessing? The theme comes up in Murakami's *What I Talk About When I Talk About Running*. After complaining about how skinny his wife is, he writes:

"But when I think about it, having the kind of body that easily puts on weight was perhaps a blessing in disguise. In other words, if I don't want to gain weight I have to work out hard every day, watch what I eat, and cut down on indulgences. Life can be tough, but as long as you don't stint on the effort, your metabolism will greatly improve with these habits, and you'll end up much healthier, not to mention stronger. To a certain extent, you can even slow down the effects of aging....We should consider ourselves lucky that the red light is so clearly visible."

He adds, wryly, "Of course, it's not always easy to see things this way." I'm here to tell you it's much easier when you feel like you're winning the struggle. But the moment you stop feeling like a victim in your skin is the moment that this whole game gets easier, so find a way to focus on the silver lining. Be grateful.

However long you run today, let it be an opportunity to explore gratitude.

JOURNAL SPACE

Write the words, "I'm grateful for the body that I have," then free associate a list of all the things you're grateful for today.

JOURNAL SPACE

Write the words, "I'm grateful for the body that I have," then free associate a list of all the things you're grateful for today.
(continued)

DAY 23:
JE NE REGRET RIEN...
EXCEPT THAT LAST GLASS OF WINE

April 27, 2010: 5.25 miles, 57:08 minutes. Maintained a steady pace and felt stronger than I did last week—no trace of alcohol in my system and primed by a few bites of leftover omelet. It does make a difference. Noteworthy: I got my mileage back up above 20 miles per week again, finally. Back in the game!

DATE: _____ TIME: _____ MILES: _____

NOTES:

So you drank too much last night. Oh no, wait a minute, that was me! But surely this will happen to you, at some point, and just because you're a friend of the bottle doesn't mean you should be denied your daily constitutional. Heck no! In fact, a run is the world's best hangover cure. Here's what to do to make it happen.

1. Sleep eight hours, no matter what. Draw the blinds, wear earplugs, don the eye mask you got last time you were lucky enough to fly to Paris—whatever it takes to get your z's.

2. Hydrate. Drink two glasses before you go to bed, and two glasses when you get up. Throw one of those vitamin-C electrolyte powders in there. You might want to go for an Alka Seltzer too, if you're really hurting.

3. Eat eggs. I couldn't tell you why, but eggs seem to be the best recovery food. Throw some ketchup on there too. You know, lycopene.

4. Drink a cup of coffee. Do this 30 minutes to an hour before your run. It clears the cobwebs.

5. Take a shower before you run. Yeah, I recommend showering before and after your run on hangover days. Get the booze grime off before you sweat out even more toxins and nastiness.

Happy running! Remember, you'll feel better after.

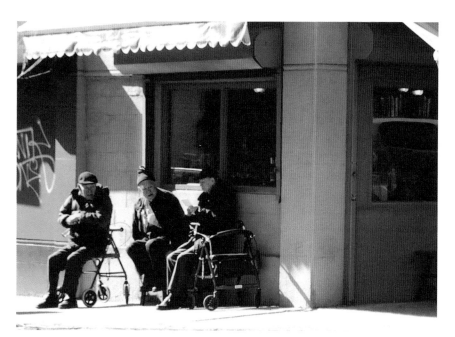

Conversation is the fountain of youth. Old men in Chinatown.

DAY 24:
SCREW THE BEAR

April 30, 2010: 2.5 miles, 27:24 minutes. YT: 289.88. I got a late start, hence the short distance, because I was writing down the story of getting flashed on the 14th St. subway platform. Proud of myself for going on a short one instead of taking an all or nothing, "I'll make up the miles later" attitude.

DATE: _____   TIME: _____   MILES: _____

NOTES:

During the Thousand Mile Year, there were many mornings that I didn't want to run. Mornings that I woke up with the energy of a hibernating bear. Becoming a "real" runner doesn't mean you spring out of bed every morning feeling like you could run and win an Olympic race. It means some mornings you're a bear, but you shrug, squeeze your paws into tennies, and run anyway.

What you'll find is that when you say, SCREW YOU, BODY, I'M IN CHARGE HERE—PUT UP AND SHUT UP, and get in even a short run, you'll go into the day and approach everything else you do with the confirmed belief that you can do whatever you set your mind to. Sweet.

When in doubt, work out!

DAY 25:
THROWING YOURSELF OVER THE LINE
May 11, 2010: 3.27 miles, 34:39 minutes. YT: 310.9 miles. Seen: An impossibly tall, willowy woman with her head shaved bald, running with the two fluffiest, squattest dogs I've ever seen.

DATE: _____ TIME: _____ MILES: _____

NOTES:

One day, about 20 minutes into my run, I realized that if I kept pace, I might be able to run 10K in under an hour, one of my goals at the time. So I did something I rarely do: I really pushed myself to the edge, physically. I made a commitment to "throw myself over the line," a friend's term for taking the leap into undiscovered country. I gave it all I had.

Alas, my finishing time for the 6.2 miles: 1:00:03. *$#$%&^%(@!!!!* Even a last-ditch sprint couldn't quite bring me in under 1:00. I hadn't given myself enough wiggle room.

So no gold-medal Hollywood ending. But I did trip at the finish line and stumble into the arms of a well-placed Ryan-Gosling look alike.

No, that's not true. But that's OK: I at least ran a quality Indie film.

Fight for your personal best. It'll feel good.

JOURNAL SPACE

Where in your life do you need to "throw yourself over the line" more often, besides running?

DAY 26:
BANISH WORKOUT BOREDOM

May 13, 2010: 5.47 miles, 1 hour, 26 seconds. Training called for 4 miles easy plus 6 x 90-sec aerobic intervals. I did them faithfully, although the last one was pretty slow because I was POOPED.

DATE: _____ TIME: _____ MILES: _____

NOTES:

At some point it happens to even the biggest enthusiast—the runner who, at first, laced up her sneakers with the gusto of a ship captain preparing his sailboat for a thrilling journey across a lusty sea. Who left for each run with a smile and a spring in her step. Who finished each run with energy to spare, already looking forward to the next.

We all get bored.

But it's easy to fix. Just mix up your training. Here's some ideas for putting new verve into your program.

1. Fartlek it. Intervals rock.

2. Try for a personal best. Sometimes we forget to challenge ourselves.

3. Alternate tempo runs with easy runs. Try 10 minutes on, 10 minutes off.

4. Reduce your mileage and throw in some weights or other cross-training.

5. Get some great new music.

6. Pick a new route.

7. Get a workout partner. I worked out with a friend today—a nice change!

8. Hit the treadmill. It will be heinous but think how much you'll appreciate your next outdoor run.

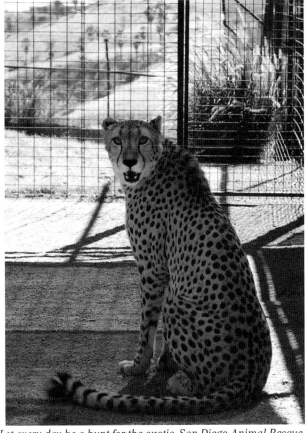

Let every day be a hunt for the exotic. San Diego Animal Rescue.

DAY 27:
KEEPING CREATIVITY FLOWING

May 15, 2010: 7.2, 1:19:24 minutes. YT: 328.17. Today I saw NY's version of LA's Kooky Groovy Lady. She was overall less kooky and groovy, but she was doing a kind of Spanish dance as part of her walk gait. It involved a lot of arm movement.

DATE: _____   TIME: _____   MILES: _____

NOTES:

"Most runners run not because they want to live longer, but because they want to live life to the fullest. If you're going to while away the years, it's far better to live them with clear goals and fully alive than in a fog, and I believe running helps you do that. Exerting yourself to the fullest within your individual limits: that's the essence of running, and a metaphor for life—and for me, for writing as well."

—Haruki Murakami, *What I Talk About When I Talk About Running*

One of the chief reasons I became a regular runner was to give my creativity a battery pack. I knew already that my brain functioned better after exercise. I knew that I had fits of creativity while on the road. But it was when I read that Haruki Murakami became a runner to keep his juices flowing that I got really excited and committed.

Murakami, who writes novels in a style that I call magical noirism, a unique blend of beauty and nostalgia, spare prose and dark, mystical conclusions, doesn't consider himself a genius. He considers himself someone who has to work hard and do everything right to continue to pump out amazing novels. He believes running saved him from being a half-baked, one-hit wonder.

And this is an important lesson: Your ability to be creative isn't just a function of the fancy or not so-fancy materials that went into your gray matter. It's equally or even more so a function of what you do with it. Do you discipline yourself? Do you intentionally create life patterns that keep your juice flowing? Do you get out of bed and run or do you slump into a heap?

Start your engines, everyone: Regularly scheduled motion is the best prevention for creative impotence.

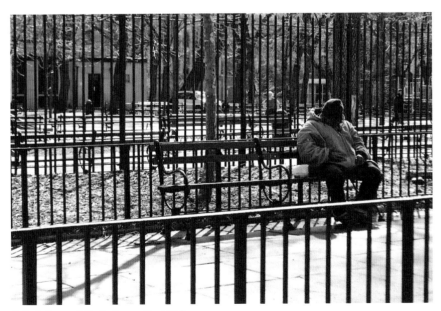

Jailed. Seward Park, Lower East Side.

DAY 28:
50 REASONS TO RUN TODAY

May 20, 2010: 5.9 miles, 1:03 minutes. Followed training plan to a T—2 miles easy, 4 x 2 min aerobic intervals, plus 2 miles easy. It felt really great to push myself on those intervals—which was excellent, because it doesn't always!

DATE: _____ TIME: _____ MILES: _____

NOTES:

There are so many reasons to run, and so few not to! Here are 35—I'm leaving it to you to come up with the final 15. You can even give yourself permission to be vain and admit you want amazing legs. I won't tell.

1. Fresh air.
2. Sexy butt.
3. Stronger core.
4. Comradery with international community of runners.
5. Opportunity to see a zillion cute dogs getting walked.
6. Mental clarity.
7. Blood sugar control.
8. Better sleep.
9. Better energy.
10. A delightfully elevated sense of well-being.
11. A sense of accomplishment.
12. Fat-melting.
13. You feel like a badass.
14. You ARE a badass.

15. Race T-shirts.
16. Sunshine.
17. Powerful legs.
18. Lower resting pulse.
19. Time to think.
20. Time to meditate.
21. Time to listen to music.
22. The knowing look other runners give you as they cross your path.
23. Improved circulation.
24. The opportunity to amuse countless friends when your foot spontaneously cramps and you shriek and jump around the room.
25. A whole new set of gadgets to obsess over.
26. Increased focus.
27. Increased patience.
28. Better sex.
29. More eating.
30. More sex.
31. Opportunities to invent stories about all the strangers who cross your path.
32. A reason to celebrate every time you hit a personal best!
33. Chocolate.
34. Chocolate cake.
35. Chocolate ice cream.

JOURNAL SPACE

Free associate 15 more reasons to run! Don't censor yourself.

36.

37.

38.

39,

40.

41.

42.

43.

44.

45.

46.

47.

48.

49.

50.

DAY 29:
HELP IN DEALING WITH CHANGE

June 10, 2010: 5.48 miles, 1:02:15 min. More speedwork today: .5m RP, .75m RP, .5 mile SP, .25m x 2 SP, .1m x2 SP, with jogging between intervals, and warm up and cool down. I really, really had to fight to crank these out, and wasn't as fast as I would have liked. I did scare quite a few squirrels.

DATE: _____ TIME: _____ MILES: _____

NOTES:

I went through a lot of change during my Thousand Mile Year. When I started, I was fresh out of a relationship, but I never expected that it would become the year that I moved from Los Angeles to New York. All that change left me feeling like a drunk person who needs to put her foot on the floor to keep the room from spinning.

One of the hardest changes was leaving my rumpled, yellow-eyed black cat in LA, because as an outdoor cat, there was only misery for him to be found in Manhattan. This cat had been my mainstay, my foot on the floor. Through three major breakups, umpteen minor ones, several jobs and a thousand different moods (both mine and his, in fact), he had never missed a meal.

To be without him was to look the reality of change squarely in the face. Thankfully, running that year offered a new constant. Looking back on it, I'm not sure how I would have survived without my 1000 mile challenge.

In the words of W.E.B. DuBois, "the most important thing to remember is this: To be ready at any moment to give up what you are for what you might become."

JOURNAL SPACE

What or who helps you flow gracefully from one change to the next? Are you relying on it/them to help you with this running challenge? You should!

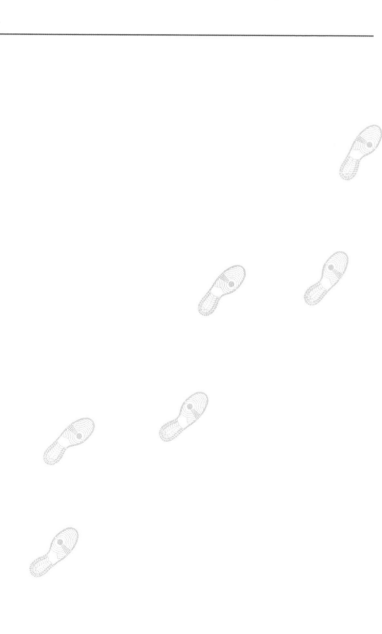

DAY 30:
SAVOR THE GIFT

June 13, 2010: 7.06, 1:15:05. Yay—awesome, awesome run!! My training called for 7 miles easy, but I took advantage of my usual energy peak at miles 4 and 5 to run them race pace, and I definitely finished strong at race pace as well, with good attention to form.

DATE: _____ TIME: _____ MILES: _____

NOTES:

Power Yoga founder Bryan Kest, in one of his early '90s videos, admonishes you, "This is your yoga for the day! Don't rush it! It's a gift! Enjoy it! Do it right!" It's almost hard to listen to him, given that he teaches the class wearing acid washed cut-off jeans and has glam-band hair. He also has a mystery accent that is most noticeable when he tells you to breathe: "*A*xhale slowly..."

Nevertheless, his words resonate.

I often hear that in my head when I run, and I say it to you now: This is your run for the day. You only get one chance to do it right. So don't fight it; make the most of the time. Savor the gift.

DAY 31:
ALICE IN BLUNDERLAND

June 17, 2010: 5.01 miles, 55:44. YT: 391.61. Decided to do a nice and easy 5-miler. The East River was steamy and beautiful today—greener than I remember, with blooming trees that smelled like honeysuckle.

DATE: _____ TIME: _____ MILES: _____

NOTES:

I learned something useful during my life's one therapy session so far. (Other than that I have trouble trusting a stranger to have useful insight into my life.)

This was it: Even good, happy events can be stressful. They are wonderful, marvelous, zoom-whee-wow—but also stressful.

I had to keep reminding myself of that as I navigated my new life in New York. Because while I'd have been an idiot not to be thankful for the twists that brought me there, I also felt like things were pretty topsy-turvy.

How does this relate to running? There will be times in your life, maybe during the 60 days of this journal, that all you can do right is crunch out a few miles. Your best made plans will disintegrate. You won't be able to strategize, or peer into your bright future. All you'll be able to do—and what you'll have to do—is get up. Get in the miles or quarter miles you can. And feel proud about it.

Hopefully that day isn't today. But when it does come, I know you'll be ready for it.

JOURNAL SPACE

You're one month in. Time to reflect: Record your successes and challenges here. If you took measurements or weighed in at the beginning, do it again today.

DAY 32:
STICKING IT OUT

June 24, 2010: 4.01 miles, 45:02. YT: 402.57. Temporary lodging at a friend's apartment in Union Square—fled from a rat in my apartment (yes, really). The morning streets of Chelsea are ruled by runners and delivery men. "Good morning track star!" one of the latter greeted me as I took off.

DATE: _____   TIME: _____   MILES: _____

NOTES:

On one of my most intense early NYC runs, I left knowing I wasn't in the best physical condition to set out for a 7-miler in the midday sun. But I decided I would anyway. I needed that cleanse of 90 minutes of motion. And I needed the miles.

In the first 20 minutes of the run, I was almost hit by a car, a tandem bike, and a kid on roller blades. At the Manhattan Bridge, I started to feel nauseated. Not so good while crossing a gigantic bridge over moving water, with subway trains hurtling by every three minutes.

Run highlight: Getting to the water fountain in East River park after three miles of dry mouth that had me staring longingly at the puddles along the water front.

A bird shat on me at mile 7.

I finished anyway.

Stick it out today, OK?

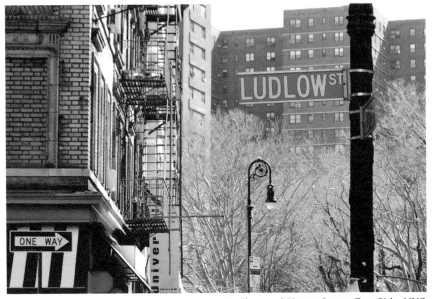

Ludlow and Hester, Lower East Side. NYC.

DAY 33:
RUNNING = AN ACTIVE CHOICE TO BE HAPPY

June 28, 2010: I only ran 1.5 this morning and didn't time it. Ninety degree heat, no air, and the noises of a new city block (new apartment!) made for a sleepless night. Ttoday's run took me into Chinatown, to the Manhattan Bridge entrance, then back down Bowery. Many smells, much activity.

DATE: _____   TIME: _____   MILES: _____

NOTES:

Things that make me happy: Sunshine. Rain. Love. Twist endings. Hugs. The freedom to make and recover from impulsive decisions.

But I also believe happiness is a state of mind. I mean, don't tell me to smile while you push me onto a bed of nails. But apart from extremes, it's more or less true. You can choose to be happy.

How do you do that? Go for your run. Screw excuses. Screw obstacles. GO. That's an active choice to be happy. It's saying, "I choose to do what makes me feel good. I choose to protect it and let everything else flow from that."

It's standing up for your belief in the best-case scenario for your life, not the rainy day version—whatever the weather.

JOURNAL SPACE

What are three simple things that you have control over that can add to your everyday happiness? Hint: One of them might be getting your run in...

DAY 34:
INTERVAL AFTERBURN

June 30, 2010: 3.6 miles, 43 minutes. Up Rivington, through the Baruch Housing complex, into East River park, up Catherine Slip, and down Bowery. This run was a little slow due to too many red lights. But I worked it with leg extensions and side bends. All in a day's run, people.

DATE: _____   TIME: _____   MILES: _____

NOTES:

Try an interval run today. High intensity interval training (HIIT) is supposed to have two benefits that are probably appealing to most everyone reading this page. First, it's supposed to lead to the fabled "afterburn," in which your metabolism stays boosted for hours after your workout. Second, it's supposed to stoke your hunger significantly less than long, steady-state runs. I fight gnawing hunger 24-7 when I'm on a heavy running cycle, but I do seem to suffer less when I do intervals. They seem to help stabilize my blood sugar.

I enjoyed this interval workout from my *Runner's World* training program and recommend you give it a try. I adapted it slightly to convert meters to miles:

1 mile warmup

.75 m at Race Pace (RP)

.5 m x 2 RP

.1 m x 4 RP

.1 m x 4 Speed pace

Between each interval, jog half the interval to recover.

DAY 35:
YOUR HAPPY PLACE

July 9, 2010: 3.92 miles, 44:54 minutes. YT: 434.11. Today I ran in the sea—not next to near, over, or beside, but IN the sea of humidity that washed over NY today. I was completely wet when I got home, and I think it was less sweat than water being pulled out of the air onto my skin.

DATE: _____ **TIME:** _____ **MILES:** _____

NOTES:

Driving on Culver toward the beach in West LA, everything changes after the stretch of warehouses when you cross Lincoln. A two-lane road cuts through the tall grasses of the Ballona Creek Wetlands. In middle June, the grass is rippled with patches that are tawny with thirst and dotted by small yellow buds. I loved driving down that road into the amniotic soup of salty, wet ocean air. It fed me.

There's nowhere I feel more relaxed than at the beach, except maybe in the ocean itself. It's the place where I feel comfortable with living and breathing, and comfortable with not breathing too. Like I could easily, painlessly be reabsorbed into what made me. I understood it when the New York artist Jeremy Blake waded into the ocean at Rockaway and never came out. Not the desire to self-destruct, but the chosen method.

Recalling a clear, vivid mental picture of your happy place can relax you when you need it by causing your brain to release oxytocin, the so-called "empathy" hormone. I know, it may be pseudo-science—but it works!

JOURNAL SPACE

Where do you feel most relaxed? Describe your happy place in visual detail to create a strong mental reference.

DAY 36:
WHAT'S A TEMPO RUN?

July 13, 2010: 3.75 miles, 51.01. YT: 443.4. A treadmill run at the Hollywood Crunch. I did intervals, from sprinting all the way down to walking. It's been a nonstop weekend of work meetings and catch ups with LA friends. Not much sleep.

DATE: _____   TIME: _____   MILES: _____

NOTES:

Let's talk Tempo Runs. More than Farklets or Interval training, tempo runs feel to me like traveling into "serious runner" terrain. Go there when you're ready.

A tempo run is a run at a continuous pace that you would consider "comfortably hard," sustained at a minimum of 20 minutes for two or three miles, if you're working toward a 5K, or four to six miles, for 10Kers.

Why would you do one? To improve cardiovascular health, but most of all, to improve your racing speed. This is how Kenyans train.

I can't say that tempo runs are very fun for me. I typically spend them wishing I were running slower. But when you're done, you feel pretty hardcore and accomplished even after just a 20-minute run.

Try pushing yourself for five minutes on one of your runs, then build in 5 minute increments.

DAY 37:
RESTRICTOR OR PERMITTER?

July 17, 2010: 10:14 miles, 2:02 hours. From the Lower East Side to the East River, around the bend to Battery Park, and up to 68th St. We walked about a mile of this, otherwise would have had a pace of around 11 min/mile. Not a bad run. Very little energy on the last couple miles, but we finished!

DATE: _____   TIME: _____   MILES: _____

NOTES:

Geneen Roth is the author of *Women, Food, and God*, one of the wisest books ever written on compulsive eating—by which I mean that you can read it and learn something about yourself and the world whether or not you have an emotionally-driven food issue.

In the book, she introduces the idea that there are two types of compulsive eaters: Restrictors and Permitters. Not only do I see she's right, but I also see that the paradigm applies to more than compulsive eating. As they say, the way you do one thing is the way you do everything, so chances are you'll see it pop up in the way you train. Meanwhile, running is a tool for taming either of these compulsive types.

"Restrictors," writes Geneen, "believe in control. Of themselves, their food intake, their environments....Restrictors operate on the conviction that chaos is imminent and steps need to be taken now to minimize its impact." On the other side are Permitters, who "find any kind of rules abhorrent...They are suspicious of programs, guidelines, eating charts...unlike Restrictors, who try to manage the chaos, Permitters merge with it." (Hello, Permitter here!)

Both of these survival mechanisms are doorways to "the euphoria of the present moment. The moment you distinguish between acting out the impulse to move away from the present moment by starving or stuffing and the awareness of the impulse to move away, you are no longer captive to your [painful] past."

You as a reader of this book might be in either camp, because "everyone is both Permitter and Restrictor. A Restrictor turns into a Permitter the moment she binges. A Permitter becomes a Restrictor every time she has decided that she is going to follow a program, even if that resolution only lasts two hours."

So, once you've identified which camp you fall in—and I think you'll know immediately which way you lean—the next question is what to do about it. The answer lies in presence, willingness to experience fully the sensations and feelings of any given moment, and to sit with them. Restrictors are usually physically self aware, but accustomed to ignoring their feelings. Permitters have used food (or other compulsions) to leave their bodies so they tend not to be used to paying proper attention.

If you feel like compulsive behavior gets in the way of your efforts, whether your diet or fitness goals, or anything else, I highly recommend you give *Women, Food, and God* a look. (God is used in a general spiritual sense; it's not a religious book.)

These are deep issues to work with over time, but your runs can be a solid training ground to practice moving toward the center, toward greater self-awareness. In fact, it's important that you do practice it, because those same compulsive behaviors can sink your program. A Restrictor might ignore her body's signals to ease off during grueling training paces, or push herself so far she falls off the wagon entirely. A Permitter might fail to recognize those signals, or start to regard their training as a restrictive activity to be avoided.

When you run, consciously check in with your body. Scan

your muscles. Explore sensation—give it words in your mind: *Achy, tight, energized, strong.* Maybe even more important, pay attention to and regulate your breath. Focus on evening out the length of your inhale and your exhale, and breathing on a count. Practice pausing between breaths.

Breath awareness is how yogis step into the present. It can work for runners, too.

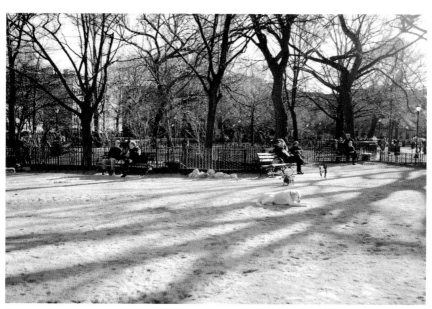

Contemplation light. Tomkins Square Park, East Village, NYC.

DAY 38:
CELEBRATE YOUR ASSETS

July 20, 2010: 5.1 miles, 57 minutes. YT: 465.58. Humid beyond belief. A storm wind blew in toward the very end; the sky darkened but didn't give any rain. I saw a man doing Tai Chi: slow and excrutiating, with a matching look on his face. Arms to held to the sky like he was shooting the sun.

DATE: _____   TIME: _____   MILES: _____

NOTES:

There came a day in my life when I realized that the men I dated didn't like me despite my gigantic rear end. They liked me because of it. My ass was an asset, for a select and celebrated subset of gentlemen.

Honestly, that was a great day, and it points toward one of the best ways to be successful, authentic, and happy. Don't change for people, or waste too much energy or angst on the ones who aren't biting.

As the Silicon Valley investor Heidi Roizen said in her interview on the Social Capitalist podcast, talking about how she dealt with sexism in tech, "My feeling was that there was always someone else I could go to. There was always another door I could open. And as many times as being a woman hurt me, it probably helped me."

Take care of your body, learn to love it, and then find those heroes who want to join your fan club, ass and all. Also recognize that of all the attributes that make you *you*, your rear end is the least important to fight for—so make sure it doesn't distract you from protecting and developing the things that really matter. A healthy, beautiful body is just a tool to help you love, create, and give back to your community.

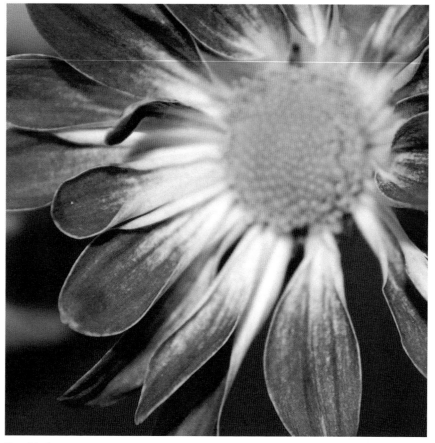

Revel in beauty.

DAY 39:
RACE AGAINST TIME

July 20, 2010: 4 miles, 46 minutes. Not much to report really. I ate two wasa crackers with feta (literally the only thing in the house) prior and felt like I could feel them kick in when I usually lose steam at two to three miles. Go power feta.

DATE: _____ TIME: _____ MILES: _____

NOTES:

Your goal: Get to the point where you feel like 25 miles of running per week is the solution to your overwhelming life, not the cause of it. Not easy for most of us.

But here's another way to think about it: There are 168 hours in a week. For me, I need to sleep eight hours a night, or life gets very confusing. That leaves me with 112 hours a week to do with as I choose.

Let's admit that at the very least, I also have 50 hours of work that must get done. Still, I have 62 hours to play with. Only five of them need to be running.

OK, I can do that. How about you?

JOURNAL SPACE

Time to run your own numbers. What activities aren't really serving your well being that you could phase out to make more time for exercise?

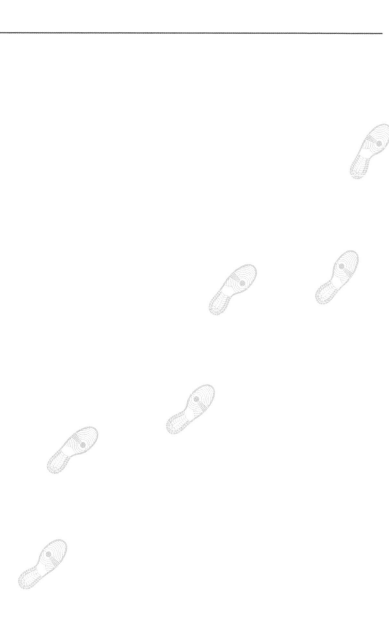

DAY 40:
WEIGHTY SIGNS—SAY, TWO TONS

July 24 2010: 5.0 miles, 53 minutes. YT: 477.08. Ah, to run on the beach! In Los Angeles for a working weekend; I had forgotten what it was like to run without immediately being in your own cloud of sweat and heat.

DATE: _____ TIME: _____ MILES: _____

NOTES:

It's not such a hard thing to run 1000 miles in a year. But it's harder when you live on a hopping, bar-packed block on the Lower East Side. It gets harder still when you happen to be a person with a natural weakness for wine and all it represents, with a minor self-disruptive tendency. Basically, there were times when the whole thing seemed pretty impossible.

And so, one day I was chewing over the question of whether to really fight for the 1000 miles, leaning towards "no." It was around October, and if I wanted to finish, I was going to have to run 25 miles a week consistently for the remainder of the year.

My friend suggested I look for a sign to guide me. Two hours later, in my usual state of oblivion to my immediate surroundings—which doesn't improve after a couple glasses of wine, which I had had—a trash truck backed into my leg while I was standing in a crosswalk. It moved slowly and stopped just exactly when it hit my leg. The only damage was a long purple bruise. If it had been going just a little faster, or stopped a little slower, I might not have run 10 miles the next day.

When I asked the universe for a sign, I was thinking more along the lines of a gentle dove fluttering past my head. Or an old lady whispering, "runnnn, Sara, runnnnnnn." Or arriving home one day, and finding that some cool company had sent me a brand new pair of running shoes, for no particular reason.

Instead, I got hit by a trash truck. And it worked. Suddenly I remembered that mobility was a gift. That week I ran 23 miles. The next week I ran more.

And that night, I did something I literally hadn't done in years: I ordered a seltzer water.

"Doing something worthwhile takes time, and training and preparation and resolve. You need to have some steel inside to see a big project through to the end." —Joel Friedlander

DAY 41:
HEALTHY DAY

August 11, 2010: 5:05 miles, 55:25 minutes. Just over 80 degrees; humidity 60 percent.
Can that really be right? I felt like I waded through this run, as reflected in my pace.
Oh well. Proud to have it done.

DATE: _____   **TIME:** _____   **MILES:** _____

NOTES:

Generally, I don't diet anymore. After years of tinkering, these days I eat fairly healthy, with tons of vegetables. But I also drink too much wine and occasionally buy soft serve from those cute little trucks. Thus I will never be slim, and am always wanting to lose five or ten pounds—mostly by the "wish upon a star" method.

Still, every so often when I'm looking to fit into my jeans, I log my foods in the free nutritional tracker at Sparkpeople.com, looking for those "hidden" calories that I down while thinking I'm Madame Svelte. It's always so instructive to see what two or three beers will do to your daily calorie count. Not to mention the slice of pizza that will be absolutely required walking home afterwards. Or, if you're living a calmer life, how those bites and tastes here and there all day add up to an extra meal. We all have places and situations that push us to somehow, quietly, almost unconsciously, slip away from our more temperate selves.

Also, running makes me preternaturally hungry, so it's helpful sometimes to check what I'm actually eating against what I "should" be eating, regardless of what my stomach is telling me.

JOURNAL SPACE

Trying journaling your food today—record your food here and then if you're feeling really curious, input it into Sparkpeople to see how the numbers add up.

DAY 42:
NEGOTIATING

August 22, 2010: 8.03 miles, 1:24:42 plus 1.56 mile cooldown. YT: 554.56. This run was almost identical in pace to my last 8-miler but my muscles and energy felt solid all the way through. Who was that Sara who yesterday had to spend the entire day in bed due to lack of energy? Screw hormones.

DATE: _____ TIME: _____ MILES: _____

NOTES:

I've mentioned the power of positive self-talk. Here was one of my conversations with my body. I hope yours are a little bit more... positive.

Me: OK, you drank an entire pot of coffee. Time to run!

Body: No.

Me: Yes.

Body: Um.... No.

Me: YES.

Body: If you wanted me to run today, you should have reconsidered white wine at lunch AND dinner yesterday.

Me: OK. I'm definitely responsible for the glass at lunch. But I think I can blame you for the dinner.

Body: You know it doesn't work that way.

Me: Sure it does. They've known since Schopenhauer that the body can act on impulses completely separate from the conscious mind.

Body: You just made that up.

Me: Yeah, it's possible. Look....We'll only run two miles.

Body: Eh.

Me: You know you'll feel better afterwards.

Body: Meh.

Me: And maybe we'll have pizza.

Body: Done.

15 minutes later, one mile in...

Body: This isn't really so bad.

Me: Hey look, people kayaking on the East River. That looks fun!

Body: You know... maybe we should run three miles? Who runs two miles anyway? We're way beyond 2-mile runs.

Me: Word.

Another mile later...

Body: OK, time to turn home if we're running three.

Me: But this is the prettiest part of the park! If we don't finish the loop, we'll miss it.

Body: Whatever.

In the home stretch...

Me: Body?

Body: Yes, Sara?

Me: I think we can blame the dinner wine on the waitress. She wouldn't quit pouring.

Body: Done.

DAY 43:
HOW FAST CAN I INCREASE MY MILEAGE?

August 29, 2010: 8 miles, 1:26: 21 min., plus .7 miles cooldown. Felt great on this run. The pace is kind of amazing given how many times I slowed down to take photos. Those little sprint bursts I've been doing really help pick up the overall pace.

DATE: _____ TIME: _____ MILES: _____

NOTES:

Mark my words, new runners, your running will take on a whole new level of enjoyment if and when you train your way up to 5- to 8-mile runs. I realize it might sound insane now, if you're still struggling to finish three or four consecutive miles. I never thought I'd enjoy (or survive) anything beyond 5K. But over time, that changed. Once I added distance, I realized that the first three miles were the worst part of my runs. It takes a couple miles for my body to say, "OK, OK, we're running!" Then it starts to get easier. So if you've never cracked three miles, start working your way up. You'll thank yourself later.

You may be wondering how fast to increase your mileage. Here's what *Runner's World* advises:

"Follow Jack Daniels' rule .... Never add more than one mile per week for each running workout you do per week. So if you run four times a week, you can add up to four miles to your weekly training. But once you add miles, you must train at the new weekly total for three weeks before adding more mileage. Devote 10 to 12 weeks to building your base to reap maximum benefits."

"Three weeks before adding more mileage" sounds awfully slow to me. According to a knowledgeable Daily Mile friend:

"There are lots of rules of thumb, but it all boils down to balancing how much stress you put on your body vs. how much rest you give it in between. The three weeks seems pretty conservative.... The Hal Higdon plans that a lot of people, including myself, use also follow the two weeks increase, one week cut back slightly rule. Works really well for me—after two weeks of increase, I'm usually feeling it, and that cut back is very welcome."

A tip around adding mileage, something that's worked for me: If you run a regular route and want to add a leg, add it on the front end, not the back. That way you get the "new" terrain out of the way right away, and afterwards, your body/mind feels like it's on that "same old route." I get a psychological boost out of it.

DAY 44:
MY FAVORITE MANTRAS FOR RUNNING

August 31, 2010: 4:05 miles, 42:46 min. YT: 570.31. I had cramps for the first two miles ... what the hay was that, body? The second two miles were decent though. Streets of Chinatown seemed weirdly empty.

DATE: _____ TIME: _____ MILES: _____

NOTES:

I love using mantras to keep myself going. Having the unbroken rhythm in your brain really helps create the same effect in your body. It can get you through extra miles when you thought you were done. Here are some of my favorites:

- You have this.
- Finish strong.
- Do this thing.
- Large and in charge.
- Go.

Hmmmn. Not very creative. Who has something better? *Ride the wild tiger?*

If you don't have any mantras yet, develop them here. They're terrific tools to silence your complaining mind and keep your body moving.

JOURNAL SPACE

Develop new mantras. Bonus points for rhymes—and please share your best mantras on the Runner's Discovery Journal Facebook page (http://facebook.com/runnersdiscoveryjournal)! I'll be there to high-five you.

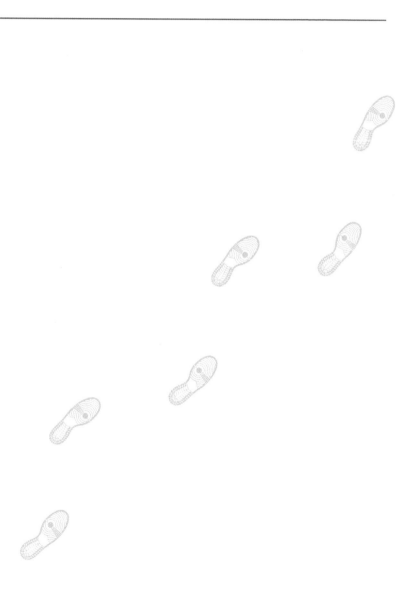

DAY 45:
INSTANT GRATIFICATION

September 23, 2010: 4.7 miles, 46:09 minutes. Post-wine runs are not nearly as effervescent as post-beer runs. I had to fight for this pace. Today I had training too: Core work, deadlifts, squats, weighted lunges, and sprints. I'm pooped.

DATE: _____   TIME: _____   MILES: _____

NOTES:

Who doesn't like instant gratification? Running has a lot to offer there: For the entire day after a good run, my body is juiced up and ready to go. I remember in high school when I first started working out, I'd end up with so much energy I'd race up and down the hallways of my house to burn it off. Those days are over, as are the days that I have a dwelling with room to run in, but the daily energy benefits of exercise are still remarkable.

But if instant gratification isn't always enough, you should also know that the long-term benefits are significant—and you don't have to be a speed demon or a distance runner to get them. In fact, some recent studies have shown that moderate running and walking have the most impact on longevity.

According to *The New York Times*, "...researchers found that running in moderation provided the most benefits. Those who ran one to 20 miles per week at an average pace of about 10 or 11 minutes per mile—in other words, jogging—reduced their risk of dying during the study more effectively than those who didn't run, those (admittedly few) who ran more than 20 miles a week, and those who typically ran at a pace swifter than seven miles an hour."

In a second study, participants "who spent one to two and a half hours per week jogging at a 'slow or average pace' during the study period had longer life spans than their more sedentary peers and than those who ran at a faster pace. This decidedly modest amount of exercise led to an increase of, on average, 6.2 years in the life span of male joggers and 5.6 years in women." And I bet the years running up to the last had a higher quality of life than they would have experienced as couch potatoes.

But studies are studies, and then there's your life. So I say run as much as makes you feel good. Just don't fool yourself into thinking that more is always better. Staying in motion over time is what matters.

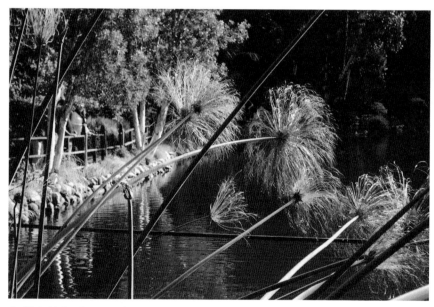

Artificial lake. Los Angeles.

DAY 46:
RED DRESS RUN

September 26, 2010: 6:43 miles, 1:08:32 in the a.m., then 3.2 miles at the Red Dress Run. YT: 662.34. WT: 27.69. Five days in a row is too many for me. I was just plain tired on my a.m. run. But I downed a beer before the Red Dress Run and was full of vim.

DATE: _____ TIME: _____ MILES: _____

NOTES:

Once I ran through Chinatown, Little Italy, and the West Village in a red dress. Actually, I was in a pack of about 80 people in red dresses. Men. Women. All in red dresses.

Why?

That's what a million smiling people asked as they snapped pictures and high fived and just plain laughed at us. And especially at the amazing bald guy in a tutu who smoked a cigar the entire run.

"Is this for breast cancer?" people asked.

"No, it's for beer," red-dress people answered. "We're anti-sobriety!"

You can read more about the distinctive tradition of hashery and its British-Malaysian roots online—in fact, Google it and see if your city has a hash. This was my first, but there will be more. In case you're thinking that it's some kind of kooky New York thing, not so. The original Red Dress Run, which attracts as many as 4500, is in San Diego, and many of those runners are Marines from Camp Pendleton. Marines love wearing red dresses. Who knew? (By the way, I got most of these details in tipsy exchanges after the run, so if any of them are wrong, I hope someday someone corrects me.)

Our route in New York was almost entirely through areas densely populated with tourists, who loved it. In Little Italy, the San Gennaro Festival was in full swing, so the streets were packed with pop-up restaurants and dense with sausage smoke. We snaked single file through the crowded streets. We must've been a column of red dresses two blocks long.

Quick summary of a hash: The leader, called the "hare," creates a trail of chalk marks showing the hashers where to run. It's full of blind alleys, as a way to slow down the people at the front of the pack and give everyone else a rest. Sometimes the trail gets lost and scouts need to be sent in all directions, looking for a mark. When it's found, everyone shouts "on on" and takes off in the new direction.

Ultimately, the hash marks lead to a bar, where everyone drinks beer, hydration be damned, and sings hashing songs.

SO MUCH FUN. Urban exploration, made-up adventure, runner's high, and drinking: A potent combination. It's silliness taken very seriously, and I love that.

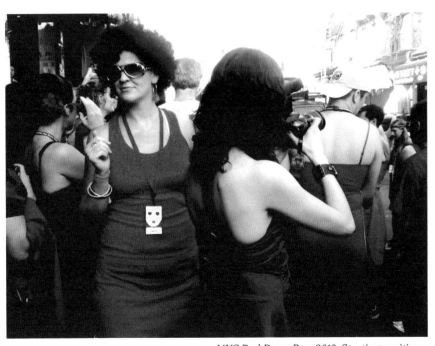

NYC Red Dress Run 2010. Starting positions.

DAY 47:
RUNNING DANCE

September 30, 2010: 4 miles, some number of minutes. This was a group hash run that started just a few blocks from my office at Madison Square and was supposed to be 5 miles. But I lost the trail at Tomkins Square Park and let myself be talked into hot-tailing it directly to the bar.

DATE: _____   TIME: _____   MILES: _____

NOTES:

A peak experience for me in the past few years was seeing Pina Bausch Dance Theatre's "Vollmond," German for *full moon*. It's a dance about romantic relationships at their most turbulent (moon-crazy), about psychic agony and sweet pleasures and emotional sturm and drang. Relationships portrayed through dance (oh God, such dance) as playful, sexy, obsessive, miserable, wonderful, manipulative, co-dependent, abusive, revelatory... but ultimately thrilling and ALIVE. And effing HOT.

That night, we all left the theatre feeling the need to spend more time dancing. I started wondering why I was spending so much time running that I could be dancing. But then today on my run, which didn't start out easy, I finally reached a moment where I broke through and went with the music, felt the chill of the October air distributed against my skin, looked up into the sun as I turned a corner and headed into an unknown street, and realized (or remembered) that running, while it may not have quite the erotic heat of dance, does open my heart to that same adventurous, exploratory state that makes me want to ROAR.

DAY 48:
TOO MUCH WINE (SUPPOSEDLY)

October 15, 2010: 4 miles, 42:00 minutes. As I was waiting for a light in Chinatown, I stretched my painfully tight quads and without really realizing it, whimpered out loud. A tiny Chinese lady with a face quilted by wrinkles smiled and chuckled.

DATE: _____   TIME: _____   MILES: _____

NOTES:

I ran 25 miles a week, worked out with a trainer, and still wasn't exactly skinny. Why? Wine. LOTS OF IT. Don't judge; it was a difficult, transitional year.

What follows was a typical conversation with my trainer at the time, who, by the way, was a slim body builder who looked like she might have weighed 120 but actually weighed 140, all muscle. She could have killed me with two fingers. Also, you have to imagine her with a French accent.

Trainer: I tell you so many times. You need to take magnesium supplements!
Me: I don't need supplements. This only happens when I drink.
Trainer: Why do you always drink before you see me?
Me: Well.... it's more like, I always drink. And sometimes I see you.
Trainer: How much are you drinking?
Me: One and a half glasses of wine, five nights a week.
Trainer: Not so bad. And you have nothing the other nights?
Me: Uh no. One I have only one. But the other I have three.

Trainer: You need to cut it. Three nights a week. Only.

Me: <cringe!>

Trainer: I mean this!

Me: <cringe!>

Trainer: OK, four nights?

Me: <nodding yes but meaning absolutely no>

Trainer: Great!

When someone French tells you that you drink too much red wine, you're in trouble.

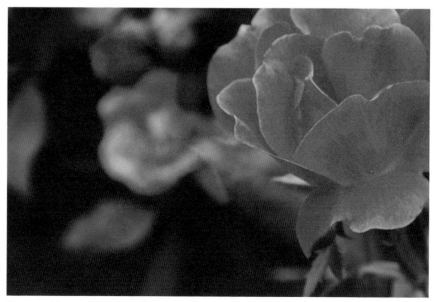

Summer Bloom. Greenport, Long Island.

DAY 49:
FINDING THE PROPER MOTIVATION

October 16, 2010: 3.14 miles, 30:17 minutes. WT: 18:85. First true cold blasts of wind. For the first time this season my long sleeve tech shirt was needed rather than hopeful. Tried to push but still landed with a less-than-exciting 9:38 pace. Looking forward to a good, long run tomorrow.

DATE: _____   TIME: _____   MILES: _____

NOTES:

Have you seen *127 Hours*, the movie about the hiker and dare devil Aron Ralston saving his life by cutting his arm off in a lonely desert canyon? It isn't an instant classic, but very well done, if you can get past the initial gruesome horror of his situation and take the journey. It's a tense one, but ultimately cathartic.

Having survived his ordeal, Aron Ralston is a motivational speaker. A quote of his I liked: "It may not be pretty, but surviving is grit and determination in its highest form. I learned that I've got the capacity to do a hell of a lot more than I thought I could if I have the proper motivation."

Today, it's your job to find that grit and determination on your run. It's better than pinning your arm under a boulder.

JOURNAL SPACE

Motivation reboot: What benefits have you experienced so far from running? How do you feel on or after your best runs? Revel in it!

DAY 50:
PLAYTIME

October 17, 2010: 8.03 miles, 1:24:15, plus .27 cooldown. YT: 729.05. WT: 27.15. The run started ominously: Something fell from the sky and landed dangerously near me—and then I ran through what seemed to be a pool of blood... then left bloody footprints down a full block of Houston.

DATE: _____   TIME: _____   MILES: _____

NOTES:

Even though my runs are slow by the rest of the world's standards, I am still almost always either pushing myself, or chastising myself for not going faster, faster, faster.

It's good to remember that runs are about play and adventure, not just self-challenge. Connect with your environment today. Explore a new route. Do a few cartwheels. Find something interesting rather than thinking about your stats.

Every run, even the shortest and the slowest, is progress—especially compared to doing nothing at all.

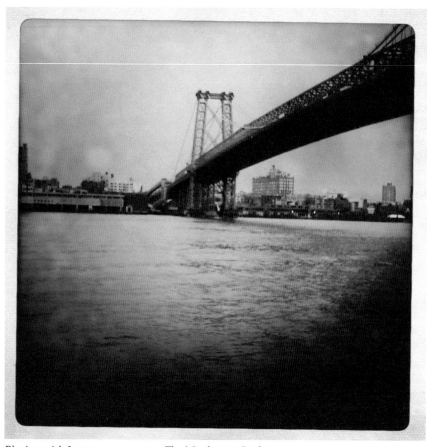

Playing with Instagram on a run. The Manhattan Bridge.

DAY 51:
RELAX TO LOVE

October 21, 2010: 4.84, 46.29. I got a very Alice in Wonderland feeling watching workmen install full-sized trees, roots covered in burlap sacks, in the concrete drag running between the Manhattan and Brooklyn bridges. "Painting the roses red! We're painting the roses red!"

DATE: _____   TIME: _____   MILES: _____

NOTES:

My dad had heart surgery toward the end of the 1000 Mile Year. It was my parents' first major health issue, and I say "parents'" beause though the physical trauma was my father's, my mother nursed him through every moment of the experience, save the operation itself.

Another *127 Hours* reference: When James Franco (as Aron Ralston) is sure he'll die and filming a goodbye video, he says something like, "Mom and Dad, I know I could have taken more time to appreciate you in my heart than I did."

There are so many people in our lives, not just our parents, who we don't take enough time to appreciate. You could spend all the time in the world with a person, and still not slow down enough to do that. We get wound so tight, we live life in a rush. We are impatient and in that impatience get brittle when what we should be is warm, open, loving, patient. Appreciating.

The brittle heart finds endless reasons not to appreciate. For example, my father calls anything with moving parts "the rotator" and gets irritated if you don't know what rotator he's referring to.

He's also in the habit of interrupting group conversations with nonsequitors. He tends to leave the door open when he goes to the bathroom, and he's prone to say things like "drop dead" when he's angry.

On the other hand, I was smiling and exchanging a few words with an elderly neighbor while walking up my stairs the other day, and I realized that one of the great gifts my father gave me growing up was the mindset that you're in a community with anyone you cross paths with. They are your friends and neighbors, whether they're older than you or younger, speak a different language, or have holes in the soles of their shoes. My father strikes up conversations with people in elevators, on street corners, in government offices. He makes everyone feel at ease, welcome and respected. During the years when he did a lot of process serves in the ghetto, they'd see him coming and whistle, "It's old blue eyes." And I always thought that was appropriate, because when he makes conversation with people, there's something lively and charming in his eyes, a kind of chuckle.

Knowing that I can connect with people the way my father does makes me feel safe wherever I go.

We have to relax to love. And I don't know about you, but I find running helps.

JOURNAL SPACE

What gifts did you receive from your parents? (Bonus if you share this with them.)

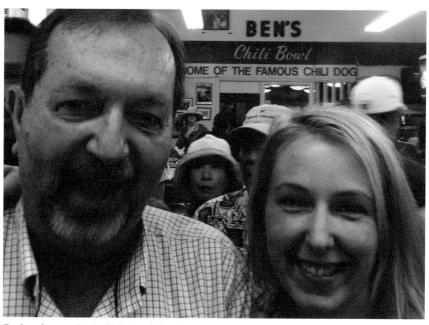

Dad and me at Ben's Chili Bowl, Washington, DC. 2011.

DAY 52:
FIND YOUR HAWK

October 22, 2010: 3.17 miles, 30:32 minutes, plus .5 mile treadmill at gym. "Pauler" (Paula, the NikePlus trainer with the Australian accent) told me that I had a personal best mile today at 9:14. Nothing else of interest to report from this shorter than usual run.

DATE: _____   TIME: _____   MILES: _____

NOTES:

There will be days that you have to do battle with the 5-year-old "I don't wanna" version of yourself. Unless you want to fight her off with a light saber, I suggest turning your run into a photo expedition. Give yourself the challenge of finding at least 10 good shots.

Consciously asking yourself to open your eyes to the world around you always yields something interesting. The first morning I tried this, that something was...

The avian John Wayne of East River Park.

I saw, and photographed, a giant hawk perched on a fence, taking one for team New York by eating a GIANT RAT. I would never have noticed it if I hadn't been on the lookout for good shots. It was the first rat I'd seen that was as big as the one in my sublet apartment (that's a story of it's own), so needless to say, in New York City, the hawk is our friend.

Like John Wayne's character in *The Man Who Shot Liberty Valance*, he's the last bastion of a wild world, taking one for the team by eating giant rats while the rest of us go to Washington and launch political careers. Or something like that. So: Take photos today. See what you see. And post the best ones on the RDJ Facebook page!

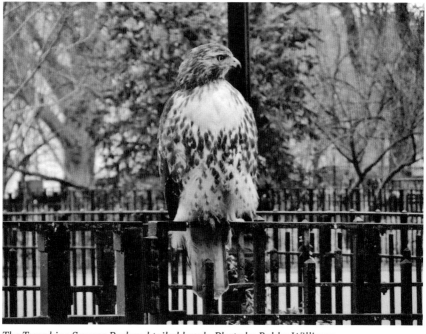
The Tompkins Square Park red tailed hawk. Photo by Bobby Williams.

DAY 53:
THREE IDEAS FOR CHANGING
UNWANTED BEHAVIORS

October 25: 2.22 miles, 20:36 min. WT: 2.22 miles. Both of my weekend runs were executed in service of other activities—picking up stuff at my office and running to a movie date with a friend, the sign of a weekend that was way too busy. So I took today off and am going to bed early to recharge for tomorrow.

DATE: _____   TIME: _____   MILES: _____

NOTES:

If you want to change the way you're doing things, "bad" behavior requires consequences.

I used to routinely skip running if I didn't have time for four or five miles. Two and three milers just didn't seem worth the schlep. Then I got to November of the 1000 Mile Year and had to institute a zero-tolerance policy around my mileage or fail. Every Saturday, I'd have to run enough distance to bring my weekly total to 25 miles— no matter what I had been up to Friday night.

Well, guess what? After a few weeks of forced 10-mile death marches, hell or hungover, I saw my future before me on those rushed weekday mornings and started gladly pulling myself out of bed for whatever distance time allowed. (Well not exactly "gladly," but out of bed anyway.)

In other words, once I instituted real accountability around 25-mile weeks, my behavior changed very quickly. It's the equivalent of cutting up your credit cards to stick to your budget; you have to know that there's no line of credit or else you keep spending.

Here are a few "consequences" that you might use to shift your behavior:

1. Set a clear-cut mileage goal like mine and do what it takes to follow through. Period. Problem is, this won't work so well if your motivation is low, so....

2. Use stickk.com to clobber yourself financially. Put $500 on finishing your desired behavioral goal, like the company's founder, the author of *Freakonomics*, did to keep his weight down.

3. Create a reward. Consequences don't have to be negative. Experiencing success (pounds melting away, new speeds reached) is one kind of reward, but these aren't guaranteed to arrive on a set schedule. So create a reward instead. Promise yourself something special if you finish—and put that something special in the hands of a committed accountability partner to dole out to you when it's due.

DAY 54:
AT YOUR CORE

November 6, 2010: 10 miles, in an amount of time I'm embarrassed to post. YT: 797.07. Still, a nice, thoughtful run, with some relaxing sadness. Another 25 mile week. Eight more to go.

DATE: _____   TIME: _____   MILES: _____

NOTES:

On today's run, think about your core values. And yes, I'm completely serious.

Every year before my birthday, I do some thinking, usually with a friend, about what I want the next year to look like. And to do that, I like to focus in on the values and concepts that animate me as a way to get to my "core" wishes. Here's what my list looked like during the 1000 Mile Year:

1. Relationships. Life's meaning is wrapped up in the connection we have to the people we care about. I want to nurture my relationships and be present in them.

2. Universality. I love to create and discover situations that strip away all the pretensions and presumptions that normally divide people. I have a strong egalitarian bent.

3. Writing. Good writing makes me giddy. I like writing, and storytelling, that digs into what it's like to be human on a very granular level—especially when the result is revelatory.

JOURNAL SPACE

What are your three core values, and how are you expressing them in your work or personal life?

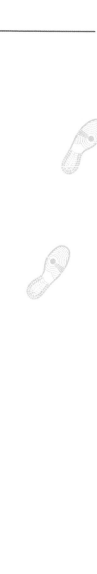

DAY 55:
LIVE THE QUESTIONS

November 11, 2010: 5.05 miles, 49:41. I went from my parents' house to the Capitol, down the mall and around the Washington Monument, and it was awesome. Sunny weather, 45–50 degrees, and a well-needed change of scenery.

DATE: _____   TIME: _____   MILES: _____

NOTES:

A favorite passage from Rainer Maria Rilke's *Letters to a Young Poet:*

"I would like to beg you dear Sir, as well as I can, to have patience with everything unresolved in your heart and to try to love the questions themselves as if they were locked rooms or books written in a very foreign language. Don't search for the answers, which could not be given to you now, because you would not be able to live them. And the point is to live everything. Live the questions now. Perhaps then, someday far in the future, you will gradually, without even noticing it, live your way into the answer."

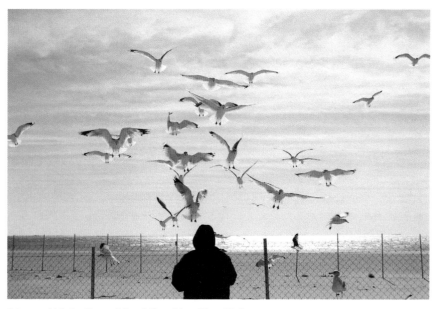

Man and birds. Coney Island, Brooklyn, New York.

DAY 56:
GETTING YOUNG WHILE GETTING OLD

November 12, 2010: 3.50 miles, 35:28 minutes; 3.56 miles, 34:46 minutes. Nothing like running home from the office with a celebratory "Remedy" gin cocktail in your belly. Actually, it was a lovely blur.

DATE: _____   TIME: _____   MILES: _____

NOTES:

The 1000 Mile Year broke my five-year track record of Inspirational Morning Birthday Runs. I strained my calf the weekend prior gallivanting around the Lower East Side on 4-inch heels.

Message from the universe: Put away childish things—not the high heels, but maybe reckless late-night gallivanting, which was no longer serving me.

That realization didn't make me feel gloomy or old. Not at all. I never feel old, not even while limping down Rivington Street wishing I had a walker. In fact, it gave me the opposite feeling. Shifting your pattern as your life changes makes you feel young.

I've always said and truly believe that the only people who really get old are the cowards to change. I always think of Matthew McConaughey's aging loser character hitting on jailbait in *Dazed and Confused*: "I keep getting older, but the girls, they stay the same age." He's old and pathetic because he's walking the same walk, year after year.

Youth requires that you keep charging forward like a toddler (or a ballerina?) into the new experiences—and opportunities—that life and maturity bring. Even those that are sobering.

And so I like to think that on that birthday, closing in on my first topsy-turvy year in New York, I was only turning 1, and fortunate to have many people to hold my arm if I toppled over.

JOURNAL SPACE

What new experiences or activities can you bring into your life to keep yourself young, playful, and exploratory?

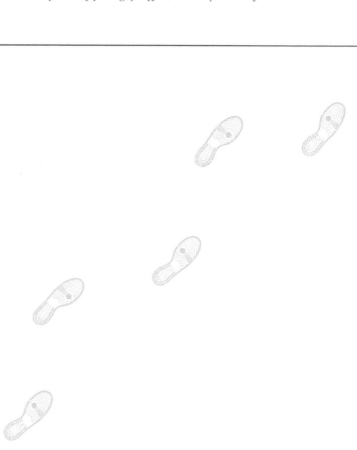

DAY 57:
DIVINITY: INTERVALS VS. STEADY-STATE
November 23, 2010: .35 miles. And 55 degrees. My birthday, and I am benched by a bum calf on a perfect running day.

DATE: _____   TIME: _____   MILES: _____

NOTES:

During the Christmas eve sermon in 2010, my parents' Episcopal priest led with a story about a Florida newspaper creating two front pages on Christmas day: one that was entirely heartwarming personal interest stories, and one that had all the bad news—a stabbing in Chicago, rebel violence in the Congo.

She appreciated that cultural impulse of the holidays, to push aside anything negative and pretend the world is only love, peace, and familial cheer. But, she said, the Christian in her was offended.

She walked us through Luke's description of Jesus' birth, with some comic annotation: "'Mary pondered,' Luke tells us. My thoughts would be similarly inappropriate for print if I was sitting in a pile of hay with my new son and a bunch of weird shepherds."

The point, however, was that there was nothing magical, warm, or fuzzy about the events surrounding Jesus' birth. Mary and Joseph were trekking to Bethlehem not to visit with family or to eat marshmallow-topped yams. They were going by decree to have their heads counted in the Roman census. There was nowhere to stay, they were hot and miserable and shacked up with sheep and strangers to birth a "surprise baby."

And yet, in all this, was the awareness of a sacred moment. The shepherds wouldn't shut up about the angels, and on some level, Mary was aware that this baby was more than merely her firstborn. This was something more.

The sermon was a gentle suggestion that we shouldn't neglect our spirit the rest of the year, amid bills and responsibilities and calamities. (The priest spoke of God's light, but let that stand for beauty, nature, humanity, as you please.) Celebrate the divine, or at least hold a space for it, even on days that are dark or dim. Life's gifts always come squeezed between life's sorrows.

Let your run nourish your spirit today.

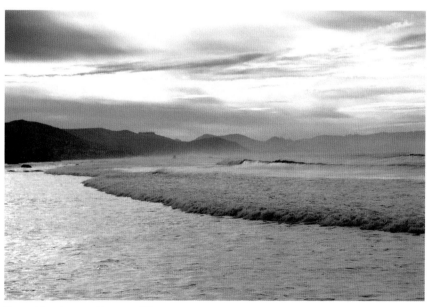

Sacred landscape. Cayucos, CA.

DAY 58:
POWERFUL AND FEARLESS

Today was two weeks to the day since my calf decided to mutiny, and I really thought I was ready. No swelling this a.m., and no pain for days, other than the very occasional twinge and some tightness. In .25 of a mile, I was proven wrong.

DATE: _____   TIME: _____   MILES: _____

NOTES:

In 1967, Kathrine Switzer became the first woman to run the Boston Marathon. When a race official tried to physically remove her from the course, her boyfriend and her coach both fought him off, and the three finished the race together.

Asked why she persisted with the training that got her to the marathon, when her university didn't even have a women's running team, Switzer told Blisstree.com, "Running is unusual: It really makes you feel very powerful and fearless and I felt really like I could do anything. I felt really like if I could run three miles a day, there wasn't anybody who could run that far."

What are you going to do with the power you cultivate in running? Run a race? Write a book? Birth a baby? Start a company?

Whatever you do, don't give up when someone official tries to spin you around by your shoulders and yank you out of the game. Know your power. It doesn't hurt to have a posse at your back, either.

And by the way, Switzer ran the race wearing lipstick. You don't have to give up every vanity to feel powerful.

DAY 59:
SEE YOU AT THE BAR

December 26, 2010: 2.23 miles, 30:14 minutes. Ran in flurries with the kind of cold that grips your throat. After three weeks of reading paleo blogs to convince myself not to eat grain, I also brainwashed myself against steady-state cardio, so this run was actually sprints mixed with walk intervals.

DATE: _____   TIME: _____   MILES: _____

NOTES:

At some point during the 1000MY, I stood in the mirror naked and took it all in. Despite many hours of morning running (followed by egg-bacon-cheese sandwiches), I really wasn't happy with the direction me ol' body had taken. I had leaned out a bit, my legs were strong, but my upper body? Not good. Clearly my lower half had been carrying my upper half all over town, like an aging dowager in a taxi. (I should have run while petting a tiny, barking Bichon on my shoulder.)

And so, I decided a little cross-training was in order. My work buddy and I signed up for personal training at the gym across the street. Let's just say, it wasn't my thing—no fun and I never felt comfortable with the expense. I had also tried to blend my old love, yoga, in with the running, and that didn't work well either—it seemed to loosen up the careful architecture my body had built to keep me in top form on the road.

It's actually just recently that I've found what I think is the perfect companion to running: The Bar Method, or any of the Lotte Burke, ballet-inspired dance workouts (Core Fusion, Physique 57, etc). The routines use isometrics and intervals to "sculpt muscles quickly" and give you a "cute dancer's butt," as founder Burr Leonard firmly tells you in her *Bar Method Accelerated Workout*. In fact, everything about Burr Leonard is firm, from her tone to the tiniest muscles of her abdomen.

I got tipped off to the Bar Method by a friend who kept posting insanely giddy Facebook status updates about how thin and toned she was getting, how great the classes were, how her sex life had been transformed.... She gave me the advice to skip past the beginning DVDs straight to the *Accelerated Workout*, and that worked for me. I also now have the *Dancer's Body Advanced Workout*. It's painful. But good.

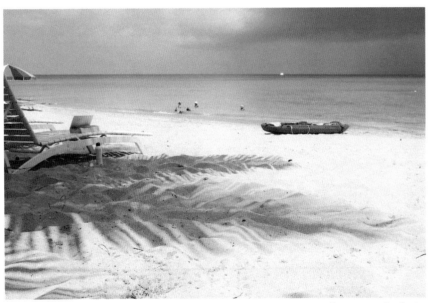

Think about paradise, not workout pain. St. Croix.

DAY 60:
SUCCESS!

December 31, 2010: 2.30 miles, 30:31 minutes. YT: 854.02. Intervals again. Warm enough to wear my 3/4 length tights, hurrah! Slush everywhere. I guess people are defrosting too: I've never had so many homeless men tell me I'm gorgeous.

DATE: _____ **TIME:** _____ **MILES:** _____

NOTES:

Congratulations! You're at Day 60!

I reached the second-to-last day of 2010, and holy moly, my 1000-mile year wasn't over! I logged 851.72 miles. In November I had been on course to finish, running 25 miles a week, but I lost three weeks to the calf injury. During that three weeks I cut carbs, lost three pounds and returned to yoga. Amazing how quickly old habits can be replaced by new habits. I think my body decided it was time for me to switch things up. It didn't care how many miles I ran.

And yet, thanks to the 1000 Mile Year challenge, I ran consistently through a move that spanned two coasts and had me living in four different apartments; through rain, snow, hangovers, and seriously stressful weeks at work. My professional efforts that year exceeded those of any year in my past, in terms of the level of my work and the fruits that it bore, and I don't think I could have done it without near-daily fitness as a constant.

Despite not finishing on time, the 1000 Mile Year project was a success—and if you're looking for a challenge beyond this journal, I highly recommend trying it. I'm living proof that you can try your hardest, fail at it, and still be happy with the results.

Thanks for spending these past months with me. This better just be the beginning for you. Running may yield to other activities. What's important is that you stay active. As long as you stay strong and fit, and keep training at something, you'll always feel like a runner now that you've become one.

Just keep putting one foot in front of the other and moving forward quickly.

JOURNAL SPACE

Did you achieve the goals you set on Day 1? What's your plan to move forward?

JOURNAL SPACE

Did you achieve the goals you set on Day 1? What's your plan to move forward?
(continued)

15440295R00066

Made in the USA
Charleston, SC
03 November 2012